Contents

D0885568

Make the best choice wherever, whenever: hundreds of foods and their *PointsPlus* values in a portable list.

A–Z Food List

The *PointsPlus* values listed here are based on nutrition information from the USDA and in some cases are an average of three different brands. Weight Watchers Power Foods are identified by a green pyramid.

A-Z Food List

▲ Weight Watchers Power Foods

A

All-fruit spread, 1½ Tbsp	1
Almonds, 23 nuts (1 oz)	5
Apple juice or cider, unsweetened, ½ cup	2
Apples	
dried, ¼ cup	1
▲ fresh, frozen, or canned without added sugar	0
▲ **Applesauce, unsweetened,** 1 cup	0
Apricots	
dried, 6 halves (¾ oz)	1
▲ fresh, frozen, or canned without added sugar	0
Artichokes	
▲ hearts	0
stuffed, 1 (7¾ oz)	15

The **PointsPlus®** values for foods in this list were current as of publication, but items may have been reformulated since then. Weight Watchers eTools, available to subscribers, may provide more up-to-date information.

▲ **Asparagus**	0
Avocado, ¼ medium (2 oz)	2

B

Bacon

Canadian-style, cooked, 1 slice (1 oz)	1
cooked, crisp, 3 slices	4

Bagel, any type

1 small	6
½ large	5

Bahamian-style peas and rice, 1 cup	9
▲ **Banana**	0
Barbecue sauce, ¼ cup	1
Barley, cooked, 1 cup	5

Note that certain foods, especially sugar-free foods, may contain sugar alcohols, which can reduce total *PointsPlus*® values. These ingredients —and also alcohol—are not typically included in food labels. As a result, you might notice discrepancies with the values you see in your lists and that you calculate with nutrition information. For the most accurate values for sugar-free foods and foods containing alcohol, please use the food lists here or in the *Shop* and *Eat Out* books,* or, if you're a subscriber, use the database on Weight Watchers eTools.

* Available for purchase at participating meeting locations

Beans, cooked

	baked, ½ cup	5
	baked, canned, vegetarian, ½ cup	3
▲	black, ½ cup	2
	black beans and rice, 1 cup	6
▲	cannellini, canned, ½ cup	2
▲	garbanzo (chickpeas), canned, ½ cup	3
▲	green	0
▲	kidney, ½ cup	3
▲	lima, ½ cup	2
▲	navy, ½ cup	3
▲	pinto, ½ cup	3
▲	refried, canned, fat-free, ½ cup	2
▲	refried, regular, canned, ½ cup	2
▲	soy, ½ cup	4
▲	wax	0
▲	white, ½ cup	3

Beef, cooked

	brisket, lean, trimmed, 3 oz	5
	chuck, arm (pot roast), trimmed, 3 oz	4
▲	filet mignon, lean and trimmed, 1 small (4 oz)	5

(continued on next page...)

Beef, cooked (continued)

▲	flank steak, trimmed, 1 slice (2 oz)	3
	ground, 95% lean / 5% fat	
▲	½ cup (2 oz)	2
▲	1 patty (3 oz)	3
	ground, 93% lean / 7% fat	
▲	½ cup (2 oz)	2
▲	1 patty (3 oz)	3
	ground, 90% lean / 10% fat	
	½ cup (2 oz)	3
	1 patty (3 oz)	4
	ground, 85% lean / 15% fat	
	½ cup (2 oz)	4
	1 patty (3 oz)	5
▲	KC strip, lean and trimmed, 1 small (4 oz)	5
▲	New York steak, lean and trimmed, 1 small (4 oz)	5
	sirloin, trimmed, 1 slice (2 oz)	3
▲	steak, lean (round or loin cuts other than those listed here with all visible fat trimmed), 1 small (4 oz)	5
	steak, regular, 1 small (4 oz)	10

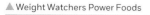
B

A-Z Food List

Beef, cooked (continued)

T-bone steak, trimmed, 1 small (4 oz)		7
▲ tenderloin, lean and trimmed, 1 slice (2 oz)		3

Beer

light, 1 can or bottle (12 fl oz)	4
regular, 1 can or bottle (12 fl oz)	5

▲ Beets   0

Biryani, chicken, 1 cup   11

Biscotti, plain or fat-free, 8 mini,
2 small, or 1 regular (1 oz)   3

Biscuits

homemade, 1 small (2½" diameter)	3
prepared from refrigerated dough, 1 small (2½" diameter) or ½ large	3

**▲ Blackberries, fresh, frozen, or canned
without added sugar**   0

**▲ Blueberries, fresh, frozen, or canned
without added sugar**   0

Bologna, beef or pork, 1 slice (1 oz)   2

Brandy, 1 jigger (1½ fl oz)   4

Bratwurst, cooked, 2 oz   5

Breads

any type other than those listed here, 1 slice	2
corn, 2" square	3
garlic, 1 slice (1½ oz)	6
high-fiber (3 g or more dietary fiber per slice), 1 slice	2
pita, any type, 1 small or ½ large (1 oz)	2
▲ reduced-calorie, any type, 2 slices (2 oz)	3

Bread crumbs, dried

plain, ¼ cup	3
seasoned, ¼ cup	3

Breadstick, 7½" x ½"   1

▲ **Broccoli**   0

Brownie, 1 (2" square)   7

▲ **Brussels sprouts**   0

Buffalo wings, cooked, 3 (4½ oz)   9

▲ **Bulgur, cooked,** 1 cup   4

Burritos

bean, 1 small (6")	7
bean, 1 large (8")	10
bean, fast food, 1 (4 oz)	6
bean and cheese, store-bought, 1 (5 oz)	7

Butter

light, 2 tsp	1
regular or whipped, 1 tsp	1

C

▲ Cabbage | 0

Cakes

angel food, 1/16 of 10" tube or 2 oz	3
pineapple upside-down, 1 piece (3 1/2 oz)	7
pound, 1 slice (5" x 3" x 1")	9
with icing, 1/12 of 9" layer cake or 3" square	14

Candies

chocolate, any type, 2 assorted pieces, 1/2 bar, or 2 Tbsp chips (1 oz)	4
hard, 1 oz	3

▲ Cantaloupe | 0

Cappuccino, 12 fl oz

▲ made with fat-free milk,* 1 tall	2
made with low-fat milk,* 1 tall	3
made with whole milk, 1 tall	3

*Counts toward a milk serving

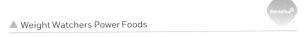
▲ **Carrots**	0
Cashews, shelled, 14 nuts (1 oz)	5
▲ **Cauliflower**	0
▲ **Celery**	0
Cereal bars	
fat-free, 1 (1½ oz)	3
regular, 1 (1¼ oz)	5
granola bar, chocolate-covered, 1 (1¼ oz)	5
granola bar, reduced-calorie, 1 (1 oz)	3
Cereals, cooked	
▲ cream of rice, 1 cup	3
▲ cream of wheat, 1 cup	3
▲ grits, corn, 1 cup	5
▲ oatmeal, 1 cup	4
Cereals, ready-to-eat	
any type other than those listed here, 1 cup	3
frosted, 1 cup	4
granola, low-fat, ½ cup	4
puffed wheat or rice, 1 cup	1
raisin bran, ¾ cup	4
shredded wheat, 1 biscuit	2
Champagne, 1 small glass (4 fl oz)	3

Cheeses

cottage

▲	fat-free,* 1 cup	3
	low-fat* (1%), 1 cup	4
	reduced-fat (2%), 1 cup	5
	regular (4%), 1 cup	5

cream

fat-free, ¼ cup	2
light, regular, or whipped, 1 Tbsp	1

feta, crumbled, ¼ cup (1½ oz)	3

hard or semisoft, dairy or soy, 1" cube,
¼ cup shredded, or 3 Tbsp grated (1 oz)

▲	fat-free*	1
	low-fat*	2
	regular	3

hard or semisoft, dairy or soy, slice

▲	fat-free,* 1 slice (¾ oz)	1
	low-fat,* 1 slice (¾ oz)	2
	regular, 1 slice (¾ oz)	2

Neufchâtel, 1 Tbsp (½ oz)	1
Parmesan, grated, 2 Tbsp	1

(continued on next page...)

*Counts toward a milk serving

Cheeses (continued)

ricotta

▲   fat-free,* 1 cup   5

      part-skim,* 1 cup   9

      whole, 1 cup   12

Cheeseburger on bun, fast food, 1 small   8

**Cheese sandwich, grilled,
restaurant type,** 1   14

Cheese twists or balls, 1½ cups   4

Cherries

      dried, ¼ cup (1½ oz)   4

▲   fresh, frozen, or canned without added sugar   0

Chicken, cooked

      buffalo wings, 3 (4½ oz)   9

      canned, with broth, ½ cup   5

      cutlet, pan-fried, 4 oz   7

      dark meat, 1 slice or ½ cup
      cubed or shredded (2 oz)   2

      nugget-style, fried, fast food, 6 pieces   9

      parmigiana, 5 oz with ½ cup sauce   11

      pieces (weights without bone)

           breast, with skin, 1 (3½ oz)   5

Chicken, cooked, pieces (continued)

▲ breast, without skin, 1 (3 oz)	3
drumstick, with skin, 1 (3½ oz)	5
drumstick, without skin, 1 (3½ oz)	4
thigh, with skin, 1 (4¾ oz)	8
thigh, without skin, 1 (4 oz)	7
salad, ½ cup	6
sandwich, grilled, fast food, 1 (7 oz)	10
sausage, cooked, 1½ oz	1
souvlaki	
1 large or 2 small skewers	5
in pita bread, 1	8

Chili con carne

without beans, 1 cup	9
fast food, 1 cup	7

Chili dog on roll, 1   11

Chili sauce, 1 Tbsp   0

Chinese brown sauce, ¼ cup   1

▲ Chinese vegetables (with peas) prepared without oil, 1 cup   2

*Counts toward a milk serving

Chinese vegetables

    with beef, 1 cup   7

    with chicken or shrimp, 1 cup   5

    with pork, 1 cup   7

    with tofu, 1 cup   4

Chocolate, 2 assorted pieces,
½ bar, or 2 Tbsp chips (1 oz)   4

▲ **Clementines**   0

Cocktail sauce, ¼ cup   2

Cocoa, hot, instant

    regular, 6 fl oz   3

    sugar-free, fat-free, 1 packet/envelope   2

Coffee, black, without sugar, 1 cup   0

Coleslaw, ½ cup   4

Conch

    cracked, 1 (6" long x 3")   10

    salad, 1 cup   3

Cookies

    chocolate chip, oatmeal, sugar,
    or similar type, 2 small (1 oz)   3

    gingersnaps, 2 small (½ oz)   2

    lace, 1 (¼ oz)   1

Cookies (continued)

rainbow, 1 (1 oz)	3
sesame seed, 2 (2" long)	4

Corn

▲ kernels, cooked, 1 cup	4
▲ on the cob, 1 medium ear (up to 7" long)	2

Corn chips, 30 small or 10 large (1 oz)   4

Cornbread, 2" square   3

▲ **Cornmeal, cooked,** 1 cup   4

Couscous (semolina), cooked, 1 cup   4

Crackers

fat-free, 7	2
matzo, 1 board	3
saltines, 5 (½ oz)	2

Cranberries

dried, ¼ cup (1 oz)	3
▲ fresh, frozen, or canned without added sugar	0

Cranberry juice cocktail

low-calorie, 1 cup	1
regular, ½ cup	2

Cranberry sauce, canned, ½ cup   6

Cream

half-and-half, 2 Tbsp	1
light, 2 Tbsp	2
▲ sour, fat-free, ¼ cup	1
sour, light, 2 Tbsp	1
sour, regular, 1 Tbsp	1
whipped cream or topping, aerosol or frozen, ¼ cup	1
whipping, heavy or light, 2 Tbsp	3

Creamer

fat-free, liquid, flavored, 2 Tbsp	1
nondairy, powder, 1 Tbsp	1

Croutons, packaged

fat-free, ½ cup	2
regular, ½ cup	3

Cuban sandwich, ½ (6½" x 3" x 4") — 12

▲ Cucumbers — 0

Currants

dried, ¼ cup (1½ oz)	3
▲ fresh, frozen, or canned without added sugar	0

D

Dairy shake, reduced-calorie, * 1 packet (¾ oz)	2
Dates	
dried, 5 (¼ cup)	3
▲ fresh	0
Doughnut, yeast, glazed, 1 (4" diameter)	6
Dressings, salad	
creamy	
fat-free, 2 Tbsp	1
reduced-calorie, 2 Tbsp	3
regular, 2 Tbsp	4
ginger, 2 Tbsp	2
Italian-type (other than creamy Italian)	
fat-free, 2 Tbsp	1
reduced-calorie, 2 Tbsp	1
regular, 2 Tbsp	2
mayonnaise-type	
fat-free, ¼ cup	1
reduced-calorie, 2 tsp	1
regular, 1 tsp	1
Duck, domestic, without skin, cooked, ¼ duck (4 oz)	6

*Counts toward a milk serving

Dumplings

potato, 6 (1" diameter)	3
vegetarian, steamed, 4 (3½" x 2")	4

E

▲ **Edamame, shelled,** ½ cup   3

Eggplant

breaded and fried, 2 slices (3" diameter)	3
▲ cooked	0
parmigiana, with sauce, 1 serving (3" x 4" with ½ cup Italian tomato sauce)	14

Egg rolls

beef or pork, 1 (4½" long)	6
chicken, 1 (4½" long)	5
shrimp, 1 (4½" long)	4

Eggs

omelet, cheese, 2-egg, 1	8
omelet, ham and cheese, 2-egg, 1	9
scrambled, 2 or ½ cup	5
▲ substitute, fat-free, ¼ cup	1
▲ whites, 3	1
▲ whole, 1 large or jumbo	2

Enchiladas

beef or pork, 2 (10½ oz)	13
cheese, 2 (9 oz)	12
chicken, 2 (10½ oz)	11

▲ Endive   0

English muffin

▲ light, any type, 1 (2 oz)	3
regular, any type, 1 (2 oz)	3

F

Fajitas

beef, 2 (9 oz)	13
chicken, 2 (8½ oz)	10
pork, 2 (10½ oz)	14
vegetarian, 2 (11 oz)	12

Falafel

in pita, 1 large pita with 4 falafel patties	13

Fish

canned, drained

anchovies, in oil, 6 (¾ oz)	1
▲ mackerel, in water, ½ cup	4

(continued on next page...)

Fish, canned, drained (continued)

▲	salmon, in water, ½ cup	4
	sardines, in oil, 5 (2 oz)	3
	tuna, in oil, ½ cup	3
▲	tuna, in water, ½ cup	2
	dried, 1 oz	2

fresh, cooked without added fat

▲	bass, striped, 1 fillet (6 oz)	5
▲	bluefish, 1 fillet (6 oz)	6
▲	carp, 1 fillet (6 oz)	7
▲	catfish, 1 fillet (6 oz)	6
▲	cod, 1 fillet (3 oz)	2
	eel, 1 oz	2
▲	flounder, 1 fillet (6 oz)	4
▲	grouper, 1 fillet (6 oz)	4
▲	haddock, 1 fillet (6 oz)	4
▲	halibut, 1 fillet or steak (6 oz)	5
	herring, 1 oz	1
	lox, 1 oz	1
	mackerel, 1 fillet (6 oz)	8
▲	mahimahi (dolphinfish), 1 fillet (6 oz)	4
▲	perch, 1 fillet (6 oz)	4

Fish, fresh, cooked without added fat (continued)

▲	pike, 1 fillet (6 oz)	4
▲	pollack, 1 fillet (6 oz)	4
	pompano, 1 fillet (6 oz)	9
▲	rockfish, 1 fillet (6 oz)	5
	salmon, farm-raised, ½ fillet (6 oz)	9
▲	salmon, wild, ½ fillet (6 oz)	7
▲	snapper, 1 fillet (6 oz)	5
▲	sole, 1 fillet (6 oz)	4
▲	swordfish, 1 fillet or steak (6 oz)	6
▲	tilapia, 1 fillet (3 oz)	2
▲	trout, rainbow, 1 fillet (6 oz)	6
▲	tuna, 1 fillet or steak (6 oz)	5
▲	whitefish, smoked, 2 oz	1
▲	whiting, 6 oz	4

Fish and cheese sandwich, fried, fast food, 1   14

Flour, whole-wheat or white, 2 Tbsp   1

French fries

fast food, 1 medium serving (4¾ oz)	11
frozen, baked, 15 (3 oz)	3
homemade, 20 (4½" long each)	11

French toast, 2 slices	8
Fruit, dried, mixed, ¼ cup (1½ oz)	3
Fruit butter, 1 Tbsp	1
▲ **Fruit salad, canned without added sugar**	0
Fudge, with or without nuts, 1 piece (1" x 2")	3

G

Garlic bread, 1 slice (1½ oz)	6
Gelatin	
▲ sugar-free, prepared, ½ cup	0
unflavored, 1 packet	1
Gin, 1 jigger (1½ fl oz)	4
Graham crackers, 2 (2½" squares) or 2 Tbsp crumbs	2
Grape juice, ½ cup	2
▲ **Grapefruit, fresh, frozen, or canned without added sugar**	0
Grapefruit juice, ½ cup	1
▲ **Grapes**	0
Gravy	
brown, ¼ cup	3
cream, ¼ cup	4

▲ **Greens (beet, chard, collard, dandelion, kale, mustard, turnip)**	0
Guacamole, ¼ cup	2
Gyoza, 3	3

H

Half-and-half, 2 Tbsp	1
Ham, cooked	
▲ lean, 1 slice or ½ cup cubed or shredded (2 oz)	2
regular, 1 slice or ½ cup cubed or shredded (2 oz)	3
Hamburger	
meat (see Beef, ground)	
on bun, fast food, 1 small	7
roll or bun, 1 (2 oz)	4
▲ **Hearts of palm (palmetto)**	0
Hibachi	
chicken, 1 cup	8
shrimp, 1 cup	6
steak, 1 cup	10
vegetables, 1 cup	5
Honey, 1 Tbsp	2

▲ **Honeydew melon**	0
Hot dog	
beef or pork	
fat-free, 1 (1¾ oz)	1
light, 1 (1¾ oz)	2
regular, 1 (2 oz)	5
on roll, plain, 1	8
roll or bun, 1 (2 oz)	4
turkey, 1 (2 oz)	3
Hummus, ¼ cup	4

I

Ice cream	
fat-free, no sugar added, or sweetened with sugar, 1 scoop or ½ cup	2
light, sweetened with sugar, 1 scoop or ½ cup	3
premium, 1 scoop or ½ cup	8
regular, 1 scoop or ½ cup	4
Ice cream cone, plain or sugar, 1 small	1

J

Jam, 1 Tbsp	1
Jelly, 1 Tbsp	1
▲ **Jerusalem artichokes**	0
▲ **Jicama**	0

K

Ketchup, ¼ cup	2
▲ **Kiwifruit**	0
Knish, potato, 1 (3½" square)	7
Knockwurst, 2 oz	5

L

Lamb, cooked	
ground, ½ cup or 2 oz	4
leg, lean, trimmed, 1 slice (2 oz)	3
loin, trimmed, 1 slice (2 oz)	3
shoulder, 1 slice (2 oz)	5
Lamb masala, 1 cup	7
Lasagna with meat, 4" x 2½" or 1 cup	7

Latte, 12 fl oz

▲ made with fat-free milk,* 1 tall	3
made with low-fat milk,* 1 tall	4
made with whole milk, 1 tall	5

▲ **Lentils, cooked,** ½ cup   2

▲ **Lettuce, any type**   0

Liquor (brandy, gin, rum, scotch, tequila, vodka, whiskey), 1 jigger (1½ fl oz)   4

Liver, cooked

▲ beef, 1 slice or ½ cup (2 oz)	2
chicken, ½ cup (2 oz)	2

Lo mein

beef, 1 cup	10
chicken, pork, or shrimp, 1 cup	9
vegetable, 1 cup	8

Lumpia (Filipino spring roll), 1 (4½" x 1" x 1½")   6

Luncheon meat

bologna, beef or pork, 1 slice (1 oz)	2
▲ fat-free, 2 oz	1
salami, beef or pork, 1 oz	3

M

**Macaroni and cheese,
package mix,** 1 cup prepared   11

▲ **Mandarin orange, fresh, frozen, or
canned without added sugar**   0

▲ **Mango, fresh, frozen, or
canned without added sugar**   0

Margarine

    reduced-calorie, 2 tsp   1

    regular, 1 tsp   1

Marinara sauce, ½ cup   3

Mayonnaise

    fat-free, ¼ cup   1

    reduced-calorie, 2 tsp   1

    regular, 1 tsp   1

Meal replacement/nutrition supplement products

    bar for weight loss, 1 (1 oz)   3

    drink,* 1 cup   6

    drink for weight loss (prepared from powder
    using fat-free milk, or canned),* 1 cup   5

*Counts toward a milk serving

Meatballs

without sauce, 2 (1¼" each) 10

with sauce, 2 meatballs and
½ cup Italian tomato sauce 13

Melba toast, 6 rounds or 4 slices 2

Milk

▲ fat-free,* 1 cup 2

instant nonfat dry powder,* ⅓ cup 2

low-fat or light (½% or 1%),* 1 cup 3

reduced-fat (2%),* 1 cup 3

whole, 1 cup 4

Milk, evaporated

fat-free,* ½ cup 3

low-fat,* ½ cup 3

whole, ½ cup 5

Milk, soy

flavored,* 1 cup 3

▲ unflavored,* 1 cup 3

Moo shoo chicken, ½ cup with 2 pancakes 8

Muffins

any type, 1 large (3" diameter) 8

store-bought, 1 large (4 oz) 12

Mushrooms

dried		0
▲ fresh		0

N

Nachos

beef, 4	14
cheese, 4 (3 oz)	9

▲ Nectarine, fresh, frozen, or canned without added sugar

	0

Noodles, cooked

cellophane, 1 cup	5
egg, 1 cup	5
fried, 1 cup	8
ramen, fresh, 1 cup	5
soba, with sauce, 1 cup	12

*Counts toward a milk serving

O

Oil

canola, 1 tsp	1
flaxseed, 1 tsp	1
olive, 1 tsp	1
safflower, 1 tsp	1
sunflower, 1 tsp	1
vegetable, any type, 1 tsp	1

▲ **Okra**	0
Olives, 10 small or 6 large (1 oz)	1
Onion rings, fast food, 1 serving (8–9 rings)	8
▲ **Onions**	0
▲ **Orange, fresh, frozen, or canned without added sugar**	0
Orange juice, 1 cup	3
Orange-grapefruit juice, ½ cup	1
▲ **Ostrich, cooked,** 3 oz	3

P

Pancake

any type from mix, 1 (4" diameter)	2
homemade, 1 (4" diameter)	3

Paneer, fried, 1 oz | 3

▲ **Papaya, fresh, frozen, or canned without added sugar** | 0

▲ **Parsnips, cooked,** 1 cup | 3

Pasta, cooked

regular, 1 cup	5
fresh, spinach, 4 oz	4
▲ whole-wheat, 1 cup	4

Pasta sauce, bottled, any type, ½ cup | 3

Pastrami

beef, 1 slice (1 oz)	1
turkey, 1 slice (1 oz)	1

▲ **Peaches, fresh, frozen, or canned without added sugar** | 0

Peanut butter, 1 Tbsp | 3

Peanuts, shelled, 40 nuts (1 oz) | 5

▲ **Pears, fresh, frozen, or canned without added sugar** | 0

Peas, cooked

▲	black-eyed (cowpeas), ½ cup	2
▲	chickpeas, ½ cup	3
▲	green, 1 cup	3
▲	snow (Chinese pea pods)	0
▲	split, ½ cup	2
▲	sugar snap	0

Pecans, shelled, 19 halves (1 oz)	6
▲ **Peppers**	0

Pickles

sweet, 1 large (3" long)	1
unsweetened	0

Pie crust, any type, refrigerated or frozen, ⅛ of 9" crust	2

Pies

fruit, one-crust, ⅛ of 9" pie	8
fruit, two-crust, ⅛ of 9" pie	11
meringue, ⅛ of 9" pie	12

▲ **Pimientos**	0
▲ **Pineapple, fresh, frozen, or canned without added sugar**	0
Pineapple juice, ½ cup	2

Pita, any type, 1 small or ½ large (1 oz)   2

Pizza, frozen

    cheese, single serving, 1   13

    pepperoni, single serving, 1   11

    sausage, single serving, 1   11

Pizza, restaurant-type, cheese

    thin crust

        1 small slice (1/8 of 12" or 1/12 of 16")   5

        1 large slice (1/8 of 16"–18")   7

Pizza, restaurant-type, one meat topping

    thin crust

        1 small slice (1/8 of 12" or 1/12 of 16")   5

        1 large slice (1/8 of 16"–18")   8

    deep-dish

        1 small slice (1/8 of 12" or 1/12 of 16")   8

        1 large slice (1/8 of 16"–18")   13

Pizza crust dough, refrigerated, frozen, or ready-made, 1 oz   2

Plantain, 1 cup   5

▲ **Plums, fresh, frozen, or canned without added sugar**   0

Popcorn

▲ microwave-popped, light, 3 cups · 2

▲ microwave-popped, plain, 3 cups · 3

▲ reduced-fat (94% fat-free), 5 cups · 3

movie popcorn, no butter, 3 cups · 4

Pork, cooked

center loin, regular, cooked, 3 oz · 4

▲ center loin, trimmed, 1 slice (2 oz) · 2

leg, trimmed, 1 slice (2 oz) · 3

loin, trimmed, 1 slice (2 oz) · 3

shoulder, trimmed, 1 slice (2 oz) · 3

▲ sirloin, trimmed, 1 slice (2 oz) · 3

▲ tenderloin, trimmed, 1 slice (2 oz) · 2

▲ top loin, trimmed, 1 slice (2 oz) · 2

Potato chips

baked, 11 (1 oz) · 3

regular, 14 (1 oz) · 4

Potatoes

baked, with vegetables
and cheese, fast food, 1 · 11

mashed, ½ cup · 3

salad, ½ cup · 8

P

A-Z Food List

Potatoes (continued)

▲ sweet, 1 large (5" long),
7 oz cooked, or 1 cup cooked — 4

white or red

▲ 1 small (1¾"–2½" diameter)
or 5 oz cooked — 3

▲ 1 medium (2½"–3¼" diameter)
or 6 oz cooked — 4

▲ 1 large (3"–4¼" diameter)
or 10½ oz cooked — 7

▲ ½ cup cooked — 2

Pretzels

Bavarian, 1 (¾ oz) — 2

rods, 2 (¾ oz) — 2

soft, 1 (2½ oz) — 6

sticks, 45 (¾ oz) — 2

twists

small, 15 (¾ oz) — 2

regular, 7 (¾ oz) — 2

Prune juice, ½ cup — 2

Prunes, 2 (¾ oz) — 1

**Pudding, from fat-free, sugar-free mix
(made with fat-free milk),*** 1 cup — 4

*Counts toward a milk serving

PQR

PointsPlus®

▲ **Pumpkin**   0

Q

Quesadilla, cheese, ½ of 6" diameter	6
Quiche, vegetable, ⅛ of 9" pie	9
▲ **Quinoa, cooked,** 1 cup	5

R

▲ **Radishes**	0
Raisins, ¼ cup (1½ oz)	3
▲ **Raspberries, fresh, frozen, or canned without added sugar**	0
Ribs (see Spareribs)	
Rice, cooked	
▲ brown, 1 cup	5
fried, with beef, chicken, pork, or plain, 1 cup	10
fried, with shrimp, 1 cup	9
Spanish, 1 cup	7
white, 1 cup	5
▲ wild, 1 cup	4
Rice cakes, plain, 2 regular or 6 mini (¾ oz)	2

Rice drinks

chocolate, 1 cup	4
fat-free, 1 cup	2
plain, 1 cup	3

Rolls

dinner, 1 (2 oz)	5
hamburger or hot dog, 1 (2 oz)	4
hard, 1 (2 oz)	4
high-fiber (3 g or more dietary fiber per roll), 1 (2 oz)	4
▲ light, 1 (1½ oz)	2

Rum, 1 jigger (1½ fl oz) — 4

S

Saag gosht, 1 cup	7
Saag paneer, 1 cup	8
Salad dressings (see Dressings, salad)	
Salads	
Caesar, 3 cups	7
chef's, without dressing, 4 cups	6
▲ fruit, canned without added sugar	0

(continued on next page...)

Salads (continued)

▲	mixed greens	0
▲	side, without dressing, fast food, 1	0
	spinach, with dressing, 2 cups	7
	taco, without shell and dressing, fast food, 1	10
	taco, with shell, without dressing, fast food, 1	18
	three-bean, canned, without oil, ½ cup	2
	tuna, ½ cup	8

▲ Salsa, fat-free   0

Saltines, 5 (½ oz)   2

Sandwiches

bagel, with cream cheese and lox, 1 large	14
cheese, grilled, restaurant-type, 1	14

Sauerkraut   0

Sausage, cooked

beef or pork, 1 link, 1 patty, or 1 oz	3
chicken, 1½ oz	1
on a roll, plain, 1 (5½ oz)	10

▲ Scallions (green onions)   0

Scotch, 1 jigger (1½ fl oz)   4

Seitan, 2 slices (2 oz)		2
Shellfish, fresh (meat only), cooked without fat		
▲	abalone, 3 oz	3
▲	clams, ½ cup (2 oz)	2
▲	crab, ½ cup (2 oz)	1
▲	crayfish, 16 (2 oz)	1
▲	lobster, ½ cup (2 ½ oz)	2
▲	mussels, ½ cup (2 oz)	2
▲	oysters, 6 medium (2 oz)	1
▲	scallops, 10 small or 4 large (2 oz)	2
▲	shrimp, 2 oz	1
▲	squid, 3 oz	2
Shumai		
	fried, 2 (2" diameter)	3
	steamed, 2 (2" diameter)	3
Soba noodles with sauce, 1 cup		12
Soft drinks, 1 can or bottle (12 fl oz)		
	club soda, unsweetened	0
	diet	0
	seltzer, unsweetened	0
	sweetened with sugar	5
Sorbet, any flavor, 1 scoop or ½ cup		2

Soups

▲	bouillon, any type, 1 cup	0
▲	broth, any type, 1 cup	0
	chicken noodle, 1 cup	3
▲	egg drop, 1 cup	1
	hot and sour, 1 cup	3
	lentil, 1 cup	4
	minestrone, 1 cup	5
	mushroom, cream of, canned (made with fat-free milk), 1 cup	5
	tomato, canned (made with water), 1 cup	3
	vegetable, 1 cup	3

Sour cream

▲	fat-free, ¼ cup	1
	light, 2 Tbsp	1
	regular, ¼ cup	3

Souvlaki, chicken

1 large or 2 small skewers	5
in pita bread, 1	8

Soy products

soybean nuts, ¼ cup (1 oz)	3
▲ soybeans, cooked, ½ cup	4
soy cheese (see Cheeses)	
soy milk	
flavored,* 1 cup	3
▲ unflavored,* 1 cup	3
soy yogurt	
flavored, ¾ cup (6 oz)	4
▲ plain, ¾ cup (6 oz)	3
tempeh (fermented soybean cake), ¼ cup (1½ oz)	2
textured vegetable protein, ⅓ cup (1 oz)	2

Soy sauce (shoyu), 1 Tbsp	0

Spaghetti, cooked

regular, 1 cup	5
spinach, 1 cup	4
▲ whole-wheat, 1 cup	4

Spaghetti sauce, bottled, regular, ½ cup	3

Spareribs

barbecued, 4 (4" long each)	9
Chinese, barbecued, 2 (4" long each)	4

*Counts toward a milk serving

▲ **Spinach**		0
Spring rolls		
	Thai, 1 (4½" long)	5
	Vietnamese, fried, 1 (4½" long)	5
▲ **Sprouts, alfalfa or bean**		0
Squash		
▲	spaghetti	0
▲	summer	0
▲	winter	0
▲	zucchini	0
Steak sauce, 1 Tbsp		0
Stir-fry		
	vegetables (with oil or sauce), 1 cup	4
▲	vegetables (without oil or sauce), 1 cup	1
	vegetables with beef, 1 cup	4
	vegetables with chicken, 1 cup	3
	vegetables with pork, 1 cup	4
Stir-fry with garlic or black bean sauce		
	beef, 1 cup	8
	chicken, 1 cup	8
	pork, 1 cup	9
	shrimp, 1 cup	7

Strawberries, fresh, frozen, or canned without added sugar   0

Stuffing mix, bread, ½ cup prepared   5

Sugar, any type, 1 Tbsp   1

Sunflower seeds, 1 Tbsp   1

Sushi

   cone, 1   3

   inari, 1   3

   maki (vegetables and rice rolled with seaweed), 6 small pieces (1" diameter x 1" thick)   3

   nigiri (sliced raw fish over rice), 4 medium pieces (1 ½" diameter x ¾" thick)   3

   nori maki (raw fish and rice rolled with seaweed), 6 small pieces (1" diameter x 1" thick)   3

Syrup

   low-calorie, pancake, 2 Tbsp   1

   regular (chocolate, maple, or pancake), 1 Tbsp   1

T

Tacos

hard or soft, fast food, 1	4
salad without shell and dressing, fast food, 1	10
salad with shell, without dressing, fast food, 1	18
sauce, 1 Tbsp	0

Taco shells, store-bought

mini, 3 (3" diameter) or ½ oz	2
medium, 1 (5" diameter) or ½ oz	2
large, 1 (6½" diameter) or ¾ oz	3

Tahini, 2 Tbsp   5

▲ **Tangerine, fresh, frozen, or canned without added sugar**   0

Taquitos

beef, 1 (5½" x 1½")	5
chicken, 1 (5½" x 1½")	3

Tartar sauce, 1 Tbsp   2

Tea, black, without sugar, 1 cup   0

Tequila, 1 jigger (1½ fl oz)   4

Teriyaki

beef, 2 slices (4 oz)	7
chicken, 2 slices (4 oz)	6
fish (other than salmon), 4 oz	6
salmon, 4 oz	7
sauce, 2 Tbsp	1
tofu, 1 cup	4

Tiramisu, 2¼" square   10

Tofu

	frozen, ½ cup	6
▲	low-fat, ⅓ cup or 3 oz	1
▲	regular, firm, ⅓ cup or 3 oz	2
▲	regular, soft, ⅓ cup or 3 oz	2

Tomatoes

▲	dried (not packed in oil), ¼ cup	0
▲	fresh or canned	0
	paste, 2 Tbsp	1
▲	puree	0
	sauce	
▲	canned	0
	Italian, ½ cup	3

Tomato or mixed vegetable juice, 1 cup	1

Tortillas

corn

½ large (10" diameter) or 1 oz	2
1 medium (6" diameter) or 1 oz	2
2 small (4" diameter) or 1 oz	2

flour

1 large (10" diameter) or 2 oz	4
1 medium (6" diameter) or 1 oz	2
2 small (4" diameter) or 1 oz	2

Tortilla chips, 12 (1 oz)	4

Tostadas

beef, 1	11
chicken, 1	10
shells, store-bought, 2	3

Tuna

canned in oil, drained, ½ cup	3
▲ canned in water, drained, ½ cup (4 oz)	2
▲ fresh, cooked, 1 fillet or steak (6 oz)	5
salad, ½ cup	8

Turkey, cooked

ground, 93% lean / 7% fat

½ cup (2 oz)	3
1 patty (3 oz)	4

▲ ground, breast, 99% fat-free

1 patty (3 oz)	3

ground, regular

½ cup	3
1 patty (3 oz)	5

▲ light meat, 1 slice or
½ cup cubed or shredded (2 oz) — 2

 ▲ Turnips — 0

Tzatziki sauce, ½ cup — 2

V

Veal, cooked

shoulder, trimmed, 3 oz	4
▲ sirloin, trimmed, 3 oz	3
parmigiana, 5 oz with ½ cup tomato sauce	13

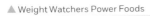

Vegetarian meat substitutes

breakfast links (sausage-type), 2 (1½ oz)	3
breakfast patty (sausage-type), 1 (1½ oz)	2
breakfast strips, 4 (1 oz)	3
burger, frozen	
patty, 1 (2¾ oz)	2
▲ patty, fat-free, 1 (2¾ oz)	2
▲ **Venison, cooked,** 1 oz	1
Vinegar, 1 Tbsp	0
Vodka, 1 jigger (1½ fl oz)	4

W

Waffles, any type, low-fat, frozen, 2 (4" round or square)	4
Walnuts, 14 halves (1 oz)	5
▲ **Water chestnuts**	0
▲ **Watercress**	0
▲ **Watermelon**	0
Wheat germ, 3 Tbsp	2
Whiskey, 1 jigger (1½ fl oz)	4
Wine, white or red (5 fl oz)	4

Y

Yam

▲ 1 large (5" long) 6

▲ 1 cup cooked 4

Yogurt

▲ fat-free, plain,* 1 cup 3

fat-free, sweetened with sugar

    flavored (vanilla, lemon, coffee),* 1 cup 4

    fruit-flavored,* 1 cup 6

▲ Greek, fat-free, plain,* 1 cup 3

▲ light (artificially sweetened),* 1 cup 3

low-fat, plain,* 1 cup 4

low-fat, sweetened with sugar

    flavored (vanilla, lemon, coffee),* 1 cup 6

    fruit-flavored,* 1 cup 7

soy yogurt

    flavored, ¾ cup (6 oz) 4

▲   plain, ¾ cup (6 oz) 3

*Counts toward a milk serving

Yogurt, frozen

fat-free

no sugar added, 1 scoop or ½ cup	3
sweetened with sugar, 1 scoop or ½ cup	3
low-fat, 1 scoop or ½ cup	3
Yogurt drink,* 1 cup	5

Z

Ziti, baked, without meat, 1 cup	7
▲ **Zucchini**	0

*Counts toward a milk serving

Seasonings and Condiments

The following seasonings and condiments have a *PointsPlus* value per serving of 0. They're perfect for spicing up foods that need a kick.

- Capers
- Extracts
- Flavorings
- Herbs
- Horseradish
- Hot sauce (pepper sauce)
- Lemon juice
- Lime juice (no sugar added)
- Mustard
- Nonstick cooking or baking spray

- Pickles (unsweetened)
- Relish (unsweetened)
- Salsa (fat-free)
- Soy sauce (shoyu)
- Spices
- Steak sauce
- Sugar substitutes
- Taco sauce
- Vinegar
- Worcestershire sauce

Great stay-in-control options,
Weight Watchers
foods and foods
endorsed by
Weight Watchers
are already
labeled with their
PointsPlus® **values.**

Weight Watchers Foods

When purchasing Weight Watchers branded products, make sure you see the *PointsPlus* logo.

Weight Watchers Foods

▲ Weight Watchers Power Foods

Weight Watchers **Baked Goods**

Blueberry Muffin, 1	4
Carrot Crème Cake, 1	2
Chocolate Brownie, 1	3
Chocolate Chip Soft Cookie, 1	2
Chocolate Crème Cake, 1	2
Coffee Cake, 1	3
Double Chocolate Muffin, 1	4
Golden Sponge Cake, 1	2
Lemon Crème Cake, 1	2
Oatmeal Raisin Soft Cookie, 1	2

Note that certain foods, especially sugar-free foods, may contain sugar alcohols, which can reduce total **PointsPlus**® values. These ingredients—and also alcohol—are not typically included in food labels. As a result, you might notice discrepancies with the values you see in your lists and the values you calculate with nutrition information. For the most accurate values for sugar-free foods and foods containing alcohol, please use the food lists here or in the *Shop* and *Eat Out* books,* or, if you're a subscriber, use the database on Weight Watchers eTools.

*Available for purchase in participating meeting locations

Weight Watchers **Bread**

▲ 100% Whole Wheat Bread, 2 slices	2
▲ 100% Whole Wheat Pita Pocket Bread, 1	3
▲ 100% Whole Wheat Wrap, 1	2
▲ English Muffin, 1	3
▲ Multi-Grain Bread, 2 slices	2
Original Bagel, 1	4
▲ Rye Flat Rolls, 1 roll	3
▲ Seedless Rye Bread, 2 slices	2
▲ Wheat English Muffin, 1	2
▲ Wheat Sandwich Roll, 1	3

Weight Watchers® By Whitman's® **Candy**

Caramel Medallions, 1 piece	1
Coconut, 1 piece	1
Crispy Butter Cream Caramel, 1 piece	1
Double Chocolate Mousse, 1 piece	1
English Toffee Squares, 1 piece	1
Mint Patties, 1 piece	1

All items in this list were current as of publication, but items may have been added, discontinued, or reformulated since then. For more up-to-date information on Weight Watchers products, please refer to weightwatchers.com/shop.

Weight Watchers® By Whitman's® **Candy (continued)**

Peanut Butter Cups, 1 piece	2
Pecan Crowns, 1 piece	1

Weight Watchers **Cheese**

Garlic and Herb Flavored Cheese Wedge, 1 wedge	1
Jalapeño Pepper Flavored Cheese Wedge, 1 wedge	1
Natural Reduced Fat Cheddar Cheese Sticks, 1 piece	2
Natural Reduced Fat Colby Jack Cheese Slices, 2 slices	2
Natural Reduced Fat Colby Jack Cheese Sticks, 1 piece	2
Natural Reduced Fat Double Cheddar Cheese Blend, ⅓ cup	2
Natural Reduced Fat 4 Cheese Italian-Style Blend, ⅓ cup	2
Natural Reduced Fat Medium Cheddar Cheese Slices, 2 slices	2
Natural Reduced Fat Pepper Jack Slices, 2 slices	2
Natural Reduced Fat Shredded Mexican-Style Cheese Blend, ⅓ cup	2

(continued on next page...)

Weight Watchers Foods

Weight Watchers **Cheese (continued)**

Natural Reduced Fat Smoked Provolone Cheese Slices, 2 slices	2
Natural Reduced Fat Swiss Cheese Slices, 2 slices	2
Natural Smoked Flavored String Cheese, 1 piece	1
Natural String Cheese, 1 piece	1
Original Swiss Flavored Cheese Wedge, 1 wedge	1
Parmesan Peppercorn Flavored Cheese Wedge, 1 wedge	1
Reduced Fat Cheese Singles, 1 slice	1
Reduced Fat Cream Cheese Spread, 1 oz container	2
Reduced Fat Onion and Chive Whipped Cream Cheese Spread, 2 Tbsp	2
Reduced Fat Pepper Jack Cheese Singles, 1 slice	1
Reduced Fat Strawberry Whipped Cream Cheese Spread, 2 Tbsp	2
Reduced Fat Whipped Cream Cheese Spread, 2 Tbsp	2
White Cheddar Flavored Cheese Wedge, 1 wedge	1

Weight Watchers **Fresh Meals**

Baked Ziti, 1 meal	5
Beef Lasagna, 1 meal	6
Beef Steak Tips in Gravy, 1 meal	5
Chicken and Mushroom Alfredo, 1 meal	6
Chicken in Curry Sauce, 1 meal	7
Chicken with BBQ Sauce, 1 meal	6
Chili Con Carne with Beans, 1 meal	5
Meatloaf with Mashed Potatoes, 1 meal	6
Roast Turkey with Stuffing, 1 meal	6
Southwestern Style Turkey Chili with Beans, 1 meal	4
Teriyaki Chicken, 1 meal	6
Three Cheese Macaroni, 1 meal	5
Three Cheese Ravioli, 1 meal	6
Turkey Meatballs with Penne, 1 meal	6
Vegetable Lasagna, 1 meal	5
Wild Alaskan Salmon Fillet, 1 meal	5

Weight Watchers **Frozen Chicken**

▲ Chicken Breasts, 1	3
Chicken Burgers, 1	3
▲ Chicken Tenders, 1	1

Weight Watchers Foods

Weight Watchers **Frozen Novelties**

Chocolate Chip Cookie Dough Ice Cream Cups, 1	4
Chocolate Dipped Strawberry Ice Cream Bar, 1	3
Chocolate Fudge Brownie Ice Cream Cups, 1	4
Cookies & Cream Ice Cream Cups, 1	4
Dark Chocolate Dulce de Leche Ice Cream Bar, 1	3
Dark Chocolate Raspberry Cheesecake Ice Cream Bar, 1	3
Dark Chocolate Raspberry Ice Cream Bar, 1	2
Divine Triple Chocolate Ice Cream Bar, 1	3
English Toffee Crunch Ice Cream Bar, 1	3
Giant Chocolate Cookies & Cream Ice Cream Bar, 1	4
Giant Chocolate Fudge Ice Cream Bar, 1	3
Giant Chocolate Fudge Sundae Cone, 1	4
Giant Cookies & Cream Ice Cream Bar, 1	4
Giant Latté Ice Cream Bar, 1	2
Giant Orange Sorbet & Ice Cream Bar, 1	3
Giant Vanilla Fudge Sundae Cone, 1	4
Giant Vanilla Ice Cream Sandwich, 1	4
Giant Wildberry Sorbet & Ice Cream Bar, 1	3
Ice Cream Candy Bar, 1	4

Weight Watchers **Frozen Novelties (continued)**

Mint Chocolate Chip Ice Cream Cups, 1	4
Peanut Butter Delight Ice Cream Cups, 1	5
Snack Size Cherry Cheesecake Ice Cream Sandwich, 1	2
Snack Size Chocolate Fudge Ice Cream Bar, 1	1
Snack Size Double Caramel Swirl Ice Cream Cone, 1	2
Snack Size Dutch Chocolate Ice Cream Sandwich, 1	2
Snack Size Vanilla Bean Ice Cream Sandwich, 1	2
Snack Size Vanilla Fudge Swirl Ice Cream Cone, 1	2
Strawberry Fruit Bar, 1	2
Strawberry Smoothie Frozen Yogurt Bar, 1	2
Turtle Sundae Ice Cream Cups, 1	5
Vanilla Ice Cream Sandwich, 1	3

Weight Watchers® **Smart Ones®**

Angel Hair Marinara, 1	6
Breakfast Quesadilla, 1	5
Broccoli and Cheddar Roasted Potatoes, 1	6
Brownie a La Mode, 1	3

(continued on next page...)

Weight Watchers Foods

Weight Watchers® Smart Ones® (continued)

Canadian Style Bacon English Muffin Sandwich, 1	6
Cheese Pizza Minis, 1 tray	7
Cheese Ravioli with Tomato Basil Sauce, 1	9
Cheesy Scramble with Hashbrowns, 1	5
Chicken & Broccoli Alfredo, 1	8
Chicken & Mushroom Florentine Smart Mini Wraps, 2 wraps	5
Chicken Carbonara, 1	7
Chicken Enchilada Suiza, 1	7
Chicken Fettucini, 1	7
Chicken in Spicy Peanut Sauce, 1	6
Chicken Marinara with Mozzarella Cheese Grilled Flatbread, 1	7
Chicken Marsala, 1	6
Chicken Mesquite, 1	6
Chicken Oriental, 1	6
Chicken Parmesan, 1	8
Chicken Quesadilla, 1	5
Chicken Ranchero Smart Mini Wraps, 2 wraps	5
Chicken Santa Fe, 1	3
Chicken Teriyaki, 1	9

Weight Watchers® **Smart Ones®** (continued)

Chicken with Broccoli & Cheese, 1	9
Chicken with Honey BBQ Sauce Smart Tortilla Rolls, 1	6
Chocolate Chip Cookie Dough Sundae, 1	4
Chocolate Fudge Brownie Sundae, 1	4
Cranberry Turkey Medallions, 1	6
Creamy Parmesan Chicken, 1	5
Creamy Rigatoni with Broccoli & Chicken, 1	7
Double Fudge Cake, 1	4
Egg Sausage and Cheese Smart Morning Wrap, 1	6
English Muffin Sandwich, 1	5
English Muffin Sandwich with Turkey Sausage, 1	6
Fettucini Alfredo, 1	6
Four Cheese Pizza, 1	10
French Toast with Turkey Sausage, 1	7
Ham and Cheese Scramble, 1	5
Home Style Beef Pot Roast, 1	4
Homestyle Turkey Breast with Stuffing, 1	6
Key Lime Pie, 1	4
Lasagna Bake with Meat Sauce, 1	7

(continued on next page...)

Weight Watchers Foods

Weight Watchers® **Smart Ones® (continued)**

Lasagna Florentine, 1	8
Lemon Herb Chicken Piccata, 1	6
Macaroni & Cheese, 1	7
Meatloaf, 1	6
Mini Cheeseburgers, 1 burger	5
Mini Rigatoni with Vodka Cream Sauce, 1	8
Orange Sesame Chicken, 1	7
Pancakes with Turkey Sausage, 1	7
Parmesan Chicken Marinara, 1	10
Pasta Primavera, 1	6
Pasta with Ricotta and Spinach, 1	8
Peanut Butter Cup Sundae, 1	4
Peppercorn Beef, 1	7
Pepperoni Pizza, 1	11
Pepperoni Pizza Minis, 1 tray	7
Raspberry Cheesecake Sundae, 1	4
Ravioli Florentine, 1	7
Roast Beef, Mashed Potatoes and Gravy, 1	6
Salisbury Steak (9 oz), 1	6
Salisbury Steak (9.5 oz), 1	7
Santa Fe Style Rice & Beans, 1	8

Weight Watchers® **Smart Ones® (continued)**

Savory Steak and Ranch Grilled Flatbread, 1	8
Sesame Chicken, 1	9
Sesame Noodles with Vegetables, 1	7
Shrimp Marinara, 1	5
Slow Roasted Turkey Breast, 1	5
Spaghetti with Meat Sauce, 1	7
Spicy Szechuan Style Vegetables & Chicken, 1	6
Strawberry Shortcake, 1	3
Swedish Meatballs, 1	7
Sweet & Sour Chicken (9 oz), 1	5
Sweet & Sour Chicken (11.2 oz), 1	9
Teriyaki Chicken & Vegetables, 1	6
Thai Style Chicken & Rice Noodles, 1	7
Three Cheese and Black Bean Quesadilla, 1	5
Three Cheese Macaroni, 1	8
Three Cheese Omelet, 1	5
Three Cheese Ziti Marinara, 1	8
Toffee Bar Sundae, 1	4
Traditional Lasagna with Meat Sauce, 1	7

(continued on next page...)

Weight Watchers Foods

Weight Watchers® **Smart Ones® (continued)**

Tuna Noodle Gratin, 1	6
Turkey Bacon Melt Quesadilla, 1	6
Turtle Sundae, 1	4
Waffles with Turkey Sausage, 1	7
Ziti with Meatballs & Cheese, 1	10

Meeting Room Products

Baked and Popped Snacks

Cheddar Twists, 1 pouch	3
Harvest Grains Cracker Chip, 1 pouch	3
Pinch of Pepper Pretzel Thins, 1 pouch	3
Popped Barbeque Potato Crisps, 1 pouch	2
Popped Chocolate Crisps, 1 pouch	2
Popped Cinnamon Swirl Crisps, 1 pouch	2

Candy and Cookies

Blackberry Fruities, 8 candies	1
Cappuccino Cream Melts, 6 candies	1
Cherry Fruities, 8 candies	1
Chocolate Swirl Mini Cookies, 1 pouch	3
Citrus Drops Jelly Candy, 12 candies	1
Ginger Snaps Mini Cookies, 1 pouch	3

Candy and Cookies (continued)

Iced Lemon Mini Cookies, 1 pouch	3
Strawberry Fruities, 8 candies	1

Drink Mixes

▲ Creamy Chocolate Smoothie Drink Mix, 1 packet (as prepared)	2
▲ Creamy Coconut Smoothie Drink Mix, 1 packet (as prepared)	2
▲ French Vanilla Smoothie Drink Mix, 1 packet (as prepared)	2
▲ Salted Caramel Smoothie Drink Mix, 1 packet (as prepared)	2

Oatmeal

▲ Harvest Berries & Cream Oatmeal, 1 container (as prepared)	3
▲ Maple Brown Sugar Oatmeal, 1 container (as prepared)	3

Snack Bars and Mini Bars

Aloha! Almond Snack Bar, 1 bar	3
Berry-licious Cashew Chew Snack Bar, 1 bar	3
Caramel Cinnamon Bun Mini Bar, 1 bar	2
Chocolate Caramel Mini Bar, 1 bar	2
Chocolate Pretzel Blast Mini Bar, 1 bar	2
Lemon Mousse Pie Mini Bar, 1 bar	2

(continued on next page...)

Weight Watchers Foods

Snack Bars and Mini Bars (continued)

Mint Cookie Crisp Mini Bar, 1 bar	2
Oh, So Nuts! Snack Bar, 1 bar	3
Praline Nut Cluster Mini Bar, 1 bar	2
Raisins 'n Honey Cereal Bar, 1 bar	3
Toasted Coconut Dream Mini Bar, 1 bar	2
Toffee Peanut Perfection Mini Bar, 1 bar	2

Heat & Eat Cups

Garden Veggie Omelette, 1 container	4
Mexican-Style Red Bean with Brown Rice, 1 container	4
Tuscan Herb & Vegetable with Whole Wheat Couscous, 1 container	4

Endorsed Products

Arnold Sandwich Thins®

▲ 100% Whole Grain, 1 roll	3
▲ 100% Whole Wheat, 1 roll	3
▲ Flax & Fiber, 1 roll	3
▲ Honey Wheat, 1 roll	3
▲ Multigrain, 1 roll	3
▲ Rye, 1 roll	3
▲ Whole Grain White, 1 roll	3

▲ Weight Watchers Power Foods

Boca® Meatless Products

All American Flame Grilled Meatless Burgers, 1 patty	3
▲ Bruschetta Tomato Basil Parmesan Veggie Patties, 1 patty	2
Cheeseburger Meatless Burgers, 1 patty	3
▲ Grilled Vegetable Meatless Burgers, 1 patty	2
▲ Ground Crumbles, ½ cup	2
Meatless Breakfast Links, 2 links	2
Original Chik'n Meatless Patties, 1 patty	4
▲ Original Vegan Meatless Burgers, 1 patty	2
Savory Mushroom Mozzarella Veggie Patties, 1 patty	2
Spicy Chik'n Meatless Patties, 1 patty	4

Brownberry Sandwich Thins®

▲ 100% Whole Wheat, 1 roll	3
▲ Honey Wheat, 1 roll	3
▲ Multigrain, 1 roll	3
▲ Whole Grain White, 1 roll	3

Green Giant® Canned Vegetables

▲ Asparagus Cut Spears, ½ cup	0
▲ Asparagus Cut Spears, 50% Less Sodium, ½ cup	0

Weight Watchers Foods

(continued on next page...)

Endorsed Products, Green Giant® Canned Vegetables (continued)

Cream Style Sweet Corn, ½ cup	3
▲ Cut Green Beans, ½ cup	0
▲ Cut Green Beans, 50% less sodium, ½ cup	0
▲ Extra Long Asparagus Spears, 5 spears,	0
▲ French Style Green Beans, ½ cup	0
▲ Kitchen Sliced Green Beans, ½ cup	0
▲ Mixed Vegetable Blend, ½ cup	1
▲ Mushroom Pieces & Stems, ½ cup	0
SteamCrisp® Chipotle Seasoned White Corn, ½ cup	1
▲ SteamCrisp® Extra Sweet Niblets® Whole Kernel Sweet Corn, ½ cup	2
SteamCrisp® Mexicorn®, ½ cup	2
▲ SteamCrisp® Niblets® Whole Kernel Sweet Corn, ½ cup	2
▲ SteamCrisp® Niblets® Whole Kernel Sweet Corn No Salt Added, ½ cup	2
▲ SteamCrisp® Southwestern Style Corn, ½ cup	1
▲ SteamCrisp® Super Sweet White Corn Whole Kernel Corn, ½ cup	2
▲ SteamCrisp® Super Sweet Yellow & White Whole Kernel Corn, ½ cup	2

Endorsed Products, Green Giant® Canned Vegetables (continued)

▲ SteamCrisp® White Shoepeg Corn, ½ cup	2
▲ SteamCrisp® White Shoepeg Whole Kernel Corn, ½ cup	2
▲ Sweet Peas, ½ cup	1
▲ Sweet Peas, 50% less sodium, ½ cup	1
Three Bean Salad, ½ cup	2
▲ Whole Kernel Sweet Corn, ½ cup	2
▲ Whole Kernel Sweet Corn, 50% less sodium, ½ cup	2

Green Giant® Frozen Vegetables

Baby Brussels Sprouts & Butter Sauce, ½ cup	1
Baby Lima Beans & Butter Sauce, ⅔ cup	2
Baby Sweet Peas & Butter Sauce, ¾ cup	2
▲ Baby Vegetable Medley, ¾ cup	1
Broccoli & Cheese Sauce, ⅔ cup	2
Broccoli & White Cheddar Cheese Sauce, ¾ cup	1
Broccoli & Zesty Cheese Sauce, ¾ cup	1
Broccoli, Cauliflower, Carrots & Cheese Sauce, ⅔ cup	2
▲ Broccoli Spears, 3 oz	0

(continued on next page...)

Weight Watchers Foods

Endorsed Products, Green Giant® Frozen Vegetables (continued)

Broccoli Spears & Butter Sauce, 4 oz	1
Cauliflower & Cheese Sauce, ½ cup	1
▲ Chopped Spinach, ½ cup	0
Cream Style Corn, ½ cup	2
Cut Leaf Spinach & Butter Sauce, ½ cup	1
Honey Glazed Carrots, 1 cup	2
Just for One Broccoli & Cheese Sauce, 1 tray	1
Just for One Broccoli, Carrots, & Italian Seasoning, 1 tray	1
Just for One Cauliflower & Cheese Sauce, 1 tray	1
Just for One Niblets® Corn & Butter Sauce, 1 tray	2
Just for One Peas & Corn in a Basil Butter Sauce, 1 tray	2
Niblets® Corn & Butter Sauce, ⅔ cup	2
Shoepeg White Corn & Butter Sauce, ¾ cup	3
▲ Simply Steam Asparagus Cuts, ⅓ cup	1
▲ Simply Steam Baby Lima Beans, ½ cup	2
▲ Simply Steam Baby Sweet Peas, ½ cup	1
▲ Simply Steam Broccoli & Carrots ¾ cup	1
▲ Simply Steam Broccoli Cuts, ½ cup	0
▲ Simply Steam Garden Vegetable Medley, ½ cup	2

Endorsed Products, Green Giant® Frozen Vegetables (continued)

Simply Steam Green Beans & Almonds, ⅓ cup	1
▲ Simply Steam Niblets® Corn, ½ cup	1
▲ Simply Steam Shoepeg White Corn, ½ cup	2
▲ Simply Steam Sugar Snap Peas, ½ cup	1
▲ Simply Steam Sweet Peas & Pearl Onions, ½ cup	1
▲ Teriyaki Vegetables, 1¼ cups	1

Jolly Time Healthy Pop®

▲ Butter, 5 cups popped	3
▲ Butter, 100 Calorie Mini Bag, 1 bag (5 cups popped)	3
▲ Caramel Apple, 5 cups popped	3
▲ Crispy White, 5 cups popped	3
▲ Kettle Corn, 5 cups popped	3
▲ Kettle Corn, 100 Calorie Mini Bag, 1 bag (5 cups popped)	3
▲ Low Sodium, 5½ cups popped	3
▲ Low Sodium, 100 Calorie Mini Bag, 1 bag	3

Oroweat Sandwich Thins®

▲ 100% Whole Grain, 1 roll	3
▲ 100% Whole Wheat, 1 roll	3

(continued on next page...)

Weight Watchers Foods

**Endorsed Products, Oroweat Sandwich Thins®
(continued)**

▲ Flax & Fiber, 1 roll	3
▲ Honey Wheat, 1 roll	3
▲ Multigrain, 1 roll	3

Progresso® Light Soup

Beef Pot Roast Soup, 1 cup	2
Chicken & Dumpling Soup, 1 cup	2
Chicken Noodle Soup, 1 cup	2
Chicken Pot Pie Style, 1 cup	2
Chicken Vegetable Rotini Soup, 1 cup	2
Creamy Potato with Bacon and Cheese, 1 cup	2
Homestyle Vegetable & Rice Soup, 1 cup	1
Italian Style Meatball Soup, 1 cup	2
Italian Style Vegetable Soup, 1 cup	2
New England Clam Chowder Soup, 1 cup	2
Roasted Chicken and Vegetable Soup, 1 cup	2
Santa Fe Style Chicken Soup, 1 cup	2
▲ Savory Vegetable Barley Soup, 1 cup	1
Southwestern-Style Vegetable Soup, 1 cup	2
Vegetable and Noodle Soup, 1 cup	1
Vegetable Soup, 1 cup	1

Yoplait® Greek 100

▲ Black Cherry, 1 container	2
▲ Key Lime, 1 container	2
▲ Mixed Berry, 1 container	2
▲ Peach, 1 container	2
▲ Strawberry, 1 container	2
▲ Vanilla, 1 container	2

Yoplait® Light

▲ Apple Turnover, 1 container	2
▲ Apricot Mango, 1 container	2
▲ Banana Cream Pie, 1 container	2
▲ Black Forest Cake, 1 container	2
▲ Blackberry, 1 container	2
▲ Blueberry Patch, 1 container	2
▲ Boston Cream Pie, 1 container	2
▲ Harvest Peach, 1 container	2
▲ Key Lime Pie, 1 container	2
▲ Lemon Cream Pie, 1 container	2
▲ Orange Crème, 1 container	2
▲ Pineapple Upside Down Cake, 1 container	2
▲ Raspberry Cheesecake, 1 container	2

(continued on next page...)

Weight Watchers Foods

Endorsed Products, Yoplait® Light (continued)

▲ Raspberry Lemonade, 1 container	2
▲ Red Raspberry, 1 container	2
▲ Red Velvet Cake, 1 container	2
▲ Strawberries 'N Bananas, 1 container	2
▲ Strawberry, 1 container	2
▲ Strawberry Orange Sunrise, 1 container	2
▲ Strawberry Shortcake, 1 container	2
▲ Triple Berry Torte, 1 container	2
▲ Vanilla Cherry, 1 container	2
▲ Very Cherry, 1 container	2
▲ Very Vanilla, 1 container	2
▲ White Chocolate Strawberry, 1 container	2

What's on the menu? Check these cuisine lists for some smart options when you're eating at a restaurant.

Dining-Out Ideas

The foods on this list have been selected because they fit nicely into the *PointsPlus*® program. Some are also Weight Watchers Power Foods.

Dining-Out Ideas

▲ Weight Watchers Power Foods

Barbecue

Baked beans, ½ cup	5
Chicken breast, barbecue, with skin and bone, 1 (4½ oz)	7
▲ Chicken breast, without skin and bone, 1 (3 oz)	3
▲ Collard greens, steamed or boiled	0
▲ Corn on the cob, 1 medium (up to 7" long)	2
Cornbread, 1 piece (2" square)	3

Caribbean

Bahamian-style peas and rice, 1 cup	9
Beans, black, and rice, 1 cup	6
Cuban rice, 1 cup	6
Curry goat, 4 oz	6
Jerk chicken breast, 1 (large breast, without skin)	5
Lechón asado (roast pork), 3 oz	4
Pigeon pea and dumpling soup, 1½ cups	9
Plantain, baked or boiled, 1 cup	5

Chinese

Beef chow mein, 1 cup	5
Chicken and broccoli, 1 cup	3
Chicken stir-fry with garlic or black bean sauce, 1 cup	8
▲ Chinese broccoli, cooked	0
Chinese roast pork, 1 cup	6
Chinese vegetables	
with beef, 1 cup	7
with chicken, 1 cup	5
with shrimp, 1 cup	5
with tofu, 1 cup	4
Dumplings, vegetarian, steamed, 4	4
▲ Egg drop soup, 1 cup	1
Egg roll, shrimp (4½" long)	4
Moo shoo chicken, ½ cup with 2 pancakes	8
▲ Rice, brown, 1 cup	5
Rice, white, 1 cup	5
Spareribs, Chinese, barbecued, 2 (4" long each)	4
Stir-fried vegetables with beef, 1 cup	4

Diner

Chef's salad, no dressing, 4 cups	6
▲ Chicken breast, without skin, 1 (3 oz)	3
Chicken noodle soup, 1 cup	3
▲ Fruit salad, canned without added sugar	0
Greek salad, without dressing, 3 cups	3
Omelet, herb or plain, 1 (2-egg)	6
Omelet, vegetable, 1 (2-egg)	8
Scrambled eggs, 2	5
Souvlaki, chicken, in pita bread, 1 (6½ oz)	8
Turkey sandwich, 1	7
Vegetable soup, 1 cup	3

Fast Food

Bean burrito, 1 (4 oz)	6
Chicken sandwich, grilled, 1	10
Hamburger on bun, 1 small	7
Pizza, cheese, single serving, 1	15
▲ Side salad, no dressing, 1	0
Taco, hard or soft, 1	4

Dining-Out Ideas

French

Bouillabaisse, 2 cups	9
Mussels marinière, 4 mussels with 3 Tbsp sauce	5
Ratatouille, 1 cup	5
Salad Niçoise, without dressing, 4 cups	9
Soufflé, cheese, 1 cup	5
Vichyssoise, 1 cup	3

Greek

Dolma, 4	5
Falafel patties, 4 (2" diameter)	8
Greek salad, without dressing, 3 cups	3
Hummus, ¼ cup	4
Shish kebab, 2 small skewers (4¾ oz)	8
Souvlaki, chicken, in pita bread, 1 (6½ oz)	8
Spanakopita, 3" square or 1 cup	9

Indian

Aloo palak, 1 cup	4
Bean and lentil stew (dal maharani), 1 cup	6
Chicken tikka, 4 oz	5
Tandoori chicken breast, without skin, 1 piece (4½ oz)	4
Tandoori fish, ¾ cup	5
Tandoori shrimp, ¾ cup	3

Dining-Out Ideas

Tip

At Applebee's,* look for these menu items, endorsed by Weight Watchers	
Cabernet Mushroom Sirloin, 1 serving	12
Creamy Parmesan Chicken, 1 serving	12
Grilled Jalapeño Lime Shrimp, 1 serving	8

Italian

Eggplant, breaded and fried, 2 slices (3" diameter)	3
Italian wedding soup, 1 cup	5
Lasagna with meat, 1 serving (4" x 2½") or 1 cup	7
Linguine with red clam sauce, 1 cup linguine with ½ cup sauce	8
Marinara sauce, ½ cup	3
Minestrone soup, 1 cup	5
Pasta, regular, 1 cup cooked	5
Pasta e fagioli, 1 cup	6
Pasta primavera, 1 cup pasta and vegetables with ¾ cup marinara sauce	7
Penne alla vodka, 1 cup pasta with ½ cup sauce	9
Pizza, restaurant-type, cheese, thin crust, 1 large slice (⅛ of 16"–18")	7
Spaghetti with marinara sauce, 1 cup spaghetti with ½ cup sauce	8
Tomato and mozzarella salad, without dressing, 2 large tomato slices with 2 oz cheese	5
Veal scaloppine, 2 pieces (4½ oz)	9
Ziti, baked, without meat, 1 cup	7

Japanese

▲ Edamame, in pods, 1 cup	3
Ginger salad dressing, 2 Tbsp	2
Gyoza, 3	3
Hibachi vegetables, 1 cup	5
Miso soup, 1 cup	2
Sushi, maki (vegetables and rice rolled with seaweed), 6 small pieces (1" diameter x 1" thick)	3
Sushi, nigiri (sliced raw fish over rice), 4 medium pieces (1½" diameter x ¾" thick)	3
Sushi, nori maki (raw fish and rice rolled with seaweed), 6 small pieces (1" diameter x 1" thick)	3
Teriyaki chicken, 2 slices (4 oz)	6
Teriyaki salmon, 4 oz	7
Teriyaki tofu, 1 cup	4

Dining-Out Ideas

Mexican / Tex-Mex

Beans, refried, ½ cup	4
Beef taco, 1 (3½ oz)	6
Black bean soup, 1 cup	2
Breakfast taco, 1	5
Burrito, chicken and cheese, 1 large (8")	8
Burrito, vegetable, 1 small (5½ oz)	6
Chicken or pork taco, 1 (3½ oz)	5
Chicken tortilla soup with cheese, 1 cup	5
Chili con queso, ¼ cup	6
Fajita, vegetarian, 2	12
▲ Pico de gallo	0
Quesadilla	
beef, ½ of 6" diameter	7
cheese, ½ of 6" diameter	6
chicken, ½ of 6" diameter	7
Spanish rice, 1 cup	7

Middle Eastern

Baba ghanoush, ¼ cup	3
Chicken shawarma, ½ cup	7
Chicken souvlaki	
1 large or 2 small skewers	5
in pita bread, 1 (6½ oz)	8
Falafel patties, 4 (2" diameter each)	8
Hummus, ¼ cup	4
Tabouli, ½ cup	6
Tzatziki sauce, ½ cup	2

Steak House

Cocktail sauce, ¼ cup	2
▲ Filet mignon, trimmed, cooked, 1 small (4 oz)	5
▲ Mushroom pieces	0
New York steak, cooked, 1 small (4 oz)	7
▲ Oysters, cooked, 6 medium (2 oz)	1
▲ Shrimp, 2 oz	1
▲ Strip sirloin, trimmed, 1 small (4 oz)	5
Steak sauce, 1 Tbsp	0

Dining-Out Ideas

Thai

Chile beef, 1 cup	7
Drunken noodles, 1 cup	6
Ginger chicken, 1 cup	8
Green curry with chicken, 1 cup	8
Hot and spicy chicken soup, 1 cup	4
Satay, without peanut sauce	
beef, 2 skewers	5
chicken, 2 skewers	3
Spring roll, 4½" long	5
Thai chicken with basil, without skin and bone, 1 breast (3½ oz)	5
Tom yum kung, 1 cup	2

Menu-Reading Help

Before you go out to eat, check this list for menu wordings that can steer you to better choices—and away from red-flag choices.

Better-choice words
- Baked
- Boiled
- Broiled
- Grilled
- Poached
- Roasted
- Steamed

Red-flag words
- Au gratin
- Battered
- Breaded
- Buffalo-style
- Buttered
- Creamed
- Crispy
- Fried
- Hollandaise
- Parmigiana
- Scalloped
- Scampi

Dining-Out Ideas

Get a handle on portion sizes to determine *PointsPlus®* values accurately.

Portion Sizes

At home it's easy to figure out portion sizes, but away from home you'll need to be able to assess portion sizes a different way. Use parts of your hand as an approximate guide.

Portion
Sizes

1 cup = fist

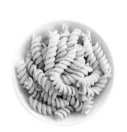

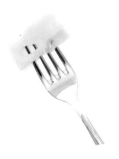

1 oz meat or cheese = thumb (tip to base)

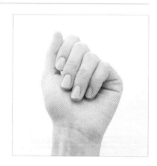

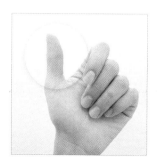

1 Tbsp = thumb tip (tip to first joint)

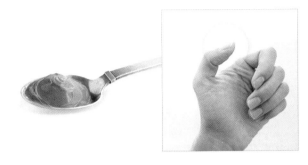

1 tsp = fingertip (tip to first joint)

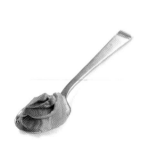
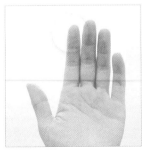

1 to 2 oz of nuts or pretzels = cupped hand

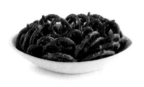 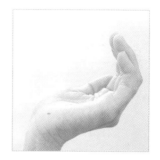

3 oz of meat, fish, or poultry = palm

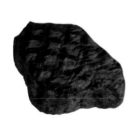 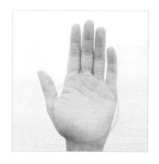

Portion Sizes

Look for the green pyramid next to foods in our lists—those are your best choices.

Weight Watchers Power Foods

Weight Watchers Power Foods are determined by both their ability to be filling (provide eating satisfaction, which keeps you fuller longer) and their impact on health (how their sugar, sodium, saturated fat, total fat, and/or fiber content stack up against that of similar foods). Foods are ranked within categories using a proprietary formula. Those that rank the highest are deemed Weight Watchers Power Foods.

Weight Watchers Power Foods ▲

Power Foods include

▲ Fruits

▲ Vegetables

▲ Whole grains

▲ Non-fat dairy & dairy substitutes

▲ Lean proteins

▲ Plus more!

An outline of what's included and what's not is listed on the follow-ing pages, but to be sure, look for the green pyramid next to foods in food lists in this *Pocket Guide* and in the *Shop* and *Eat Out* books (available for purchase in participating meeting locations). The database on weightwatchers.com (for eTools subscribers only) also indicates Weight Watchers Power Foods with pyramids.

▲ Fruits

**Need a sweet snack? Want to add something
special to a meal? With a 0 *PointsPlus*® value, fruit
is a perfect choice.**

Included
- ▲ All fresh, frozen, or canned without added sugar
- ▲ Fruit canned in its own juice (drained)
- ▲ Fruit salad—mixed fruits with no added sugar

Not included
- Dried fruits
- Juices

▲ Vegetables

Bummed by small portions? Bulk up with veggies! Most have a 0 *PointsPlus* value per serving.

Included

▲ Most fresh, frozen, or canned without added sugar or oil—whether or not it has a ***PointsPlus*** value per serving

▲ Potatoes—white, red, and sweet

Not included

- Juices
- Vegetables prepared with ingredients that are not Weight Watchers Power Foods (for example, corn in butter sauce, dried tomatoes packed in oil)
- Avocados
- French fries
- Olives
- Plantains
- Pickled vegetables

Weight Watchers Power Foods

▲ Whole Grains

Whenever you can, go for whole grains instead of refined, white grains.

Included

▲ Brown and wild rices

▲ Hot cereals, cooked—without added sugar, dried fruits, or nuts
  - ▲ 100% bran
  - ▲ Cream of rice
  - ▲ Cream of wheat
  - ▲ Grits
  - ▲ Oatmeal

▲ Pasta, whole-wheat or other whole-grain varieties

▲ Popcorn, as long as it's plain air-popped, plain or light microwave-popped, or 94% fat-free micro-wave-popped

▲ Whole-grain, ready-to-eat cereals—without added sugar, dried fruits, or nuts, and with 4 g fiber or more per serving

▲ Whole grains, such as:
  - ▲ Barley
  - ▲ Buckwheat
  - ▲ Bulgur
  - ▲ Cornmeal (polenta)
  - ▲ Whole-wheat couscous
  - ▲ Quinoa

▲ Non-Fat Dairy & Dairy Substitutes

Milks, cheeses, and yogurts are delicious, satisfying additions to meals and snacks.

Included

▲ Fat-free cheeses, including fat-free cottage cheese

▲ Fat-free milk and beverages made with fat-free milk, such as:

    ▲ Cappuccino or latte, as long as it's sugar-free

▲ Yogurt, fat-free, plain or flavored with artificial sweetener

▲ Fat-free sour cream

▲ Unflavored fat-free soy cheese

▲ Unflavored soy milk and soy yogurt

Weight Watchers Power Foods

▲ Lean Proteins

Round out meals with your favorite proteins—meats, meat substitutes, and legumes.

Included
(See food list for specific cuts and grinds)

▲ Beans, dried, and canned, including black, cannellini, kidney, refried, and white

▲ Beef, chicken, lamb, pork, turkey, and veal: lean, trimmed, and all skin removed

▲ Dried peas, including black-eyed peas and split peas

▲ Eggs: whole, whites, and egg substitute

▲ Game meats, including buffalo, ostrich, and venison

▲ Lentils

▲ Meat substitutes, including tofu and vegetarian burgers with 2 g of fat or less

▲ Most fish and shellfish: fresh, frozen, and canned in water

▲ Organ meats from beef, lamb, pork, and veal

Not included
• Canned fish or shellfish packed in oil
• Meats or fish with breading or added fat
• Processed meats, such as hot dogs

▲ Plus More!

A few foods in other categories made the cut, too.

Included breads
(Whole grains make the best choices)

▲ Light English muffins

▲ Light hot dog and hamburger rolls

▲ Reduced-calorie (light) breads or rolls, and sandwich thins

Included soups

▲ Broth, onion, and some broth- and tomato-based vegetable soups

Included desserts

▲ Sugar-free gelatin

Weight Watchers Power Foods

Build your day's eating around healthy foods, using the direction provided by these Guidelines.

Good Health Guidelines

People often ask: "But what should I eat each day for good health?" The answer lies in our Good Health Guidelines—easy advice that will help you structure your daily choices around giving your body what it needs.

Specifics about the Good Health Guidelines start on the following page and are outlined in greater detail in *Frequently Asked Questions*.

Good
Health
Guidelines

The Guidelines at a glance

Eat Weight Watchers Power Foods

- Fruits and veggies— fresh, frozen, or canned without added sugar
- Lean proteins
- Non-fat and low-fat dairy*
- Whole grains

Have Daily

- Liquids
- Healthy oils
- Multivitamin

Also Remember

- Watch your intake of:
  sodium, added sugar, and alcohol

* Non-fat options are Weight Watchers Power Foods and are better for weight loss.

▲ Eat Weight Watchers Power Foods

Weight Watchers Power Foods are the best-for-you foods. You can always find them by looking for the pyramid.

Fruits and veggies

Try to get 5 servings of fruits and vegetables per day (9 if you weigh more than 350 pounds) to help ensure you're getting enough fiber and benefiting from all the vitamins, minerals, and other natural substances found in plants.

Lean proteins

Have lean proteins each day (aim to eat 1 to 2 servings) to help stay satisfied longer and to obtain necessary amino acids, iron, zinc, and other nutrients.

Non-fat and low-fat dairy

Include at least 2 servings of non-fat or low-fat milk or other dairy products (3 if you're a nursing mom or a teenager, if you're over 50, or if you weigh more than 250 pounds) for calcium, vitamin D, zinc, phosphorus, and a raft of other essential vitamins and minerals. Note that non-fat options are Weight Watchers Power Foods and better for weight loss.

Whole grains

Select whole grains whenever possible over refined, white grains. They're rich with nutrients and fiber.

Have Daily

In addition to a focus on Weight Watchers Power Foods, each day has three to-dos.

Liquids

Make sure you're drinking 6 nonalcoholic beverages a day.

Healthy oils

Include 2 teaspoons per day of healthy oils like olive, canola, sunflower, safflower, or flaxseed (1 ***PointsPlus***® value per teaspoon), so that you get vitamin E and essential fatty acids.

Multivitamin

Take a multivitamin each day.

Also Remember

Watch your intake of added sugar and sodium. Also, limit alcoholic beverages—women should have no more than 1 alcoholic beverage each day, and men should have no more than 2.

These lists will help you decide what to buy, to make your home a weight-loss-friendly Space.

Aisle-by-Aisle Shopping Guide

Use this supermarket-friendly guide to make smart choices as you shop for your weight and for your health.

Aisle-by-Aisle Shopping Guide

Produce

Look for

- The freshest produce for the most nutrition
- A variety of colors for the widest array of vitamins and minerals
- Fruits that make good portable snacks

Tips

- Each week, try something new
- If precleaned and sliced produce will help you eat more fruits and vegetables, they're worth the expense
- Choose in-season produce for the best value and nutrition

Meat, Poultry, and Fish

Look for

- Round or loin cuts of beef; "select" grades have the least fat
- Loin or leg cuts of pork and lamb
- Boneless, skinless chicken breasts
- Lean ground turkey or ground chicken breast
- Salmon, a great source of omega-3 fatty acids, which are linked with good health

Watch for

- Combination packages of ground meats, which may not use lean cuts
- Meats prepared with marinades or stuffing. It's hard to tell how they're made

Tips

- Check the sell-by date to make sure you're buying the freshest meat possible
- Freeze if you're not going to use within a day or two of the sell-by date
- Choose fresh fish that is low in mercury, including shrimp, salmon, pollack, and catfish

Dairy

Look for
- Low-fat or fat-free versions of milk, yogurt, and cheese
- The words "live and active cultures" on yogurt containers to make sure you're taking advantage of good bacteria

Watch for
- In yogurt: added sugar, which can bump up its *PointsPlus*® value

Tips
- Choose Greek-style fat-free yogurt for a richer, less-sweet version
- Buy plain fat-free yogurt and sweeten with chopped fresh fruit
- Opt for large store-brand containers of dairy products; they are usually the best value

Deli

Look for
- Light or 99% fat-free and low-sodium packaged deli meats
- Low-fat varieties of sliced cheese

Watch for
- Bologna, liverwurst, and salami, which tend to be high in fat and sodium

Tips
- Use deli meats within two to three days of purchase, as they spoil quickly
- Divide up and freeze smaller portions if you're not going to use within three days
- To reduce sodium intake, limit your consumption of deli meats to once or twice per week

Pasta and Pasta Sauces

Look for
- Whole-grain varieties of pasta instead of regular
- Tomato-based pasta sauces, preferably labeled "low-fat" or "fat-free"

Watch for
- Pasta and sauce or seasoning combinations with added fat, sugar, or salt
- Creamy pasta sauces such as Alfredo, which have added fat

Tips
- Experiment with pastas made from brown rice or buckwheat
- If you're not ready for 100% whole grains, start with blends

Grains and Beans

Look for

- Brown and wild rice instead of regular white
- Barley, buckwheat, quinoa, and wheatberries
- Beans, peas, and lentils, which are excellent and budget-friendly sources of nutrition
- Canned beans, if time is an issue (dried beans require additional cooking time)

Watch for

- Sodium levels in packaged grain and bean mixes; choose the products that provide the least sodium per serving

Tips

- In packaged grain-based side dishes, omit the oil or butter called for in preparation—you won't miss the added fat
- Cook brown rice or other grains in low-sodium, fat-free chicken broth for added flavor
- Rinse canned beans under cold running water before you use them to reduce sodium content

Canned Goods

Look for

- Canned vegetables, a great source of nutrients and excellent for bulking up homemade soups and stews
- Fruit canned in water or juice (not in syrup)
- Tuna canned in water instead of oil

Watch for

- Added sugar or salt—check the label and opt for no added ingredients

Tips

- Rinse canned vegetables in running water before use to reduce sodium content
- Add canned vegetables to pasta sauces for added bulk with few calories
- Add canned vegetables to soups, stews, and chilis to add volume
- Choose canned fish that is lower in mercury, including shrimp, light tuna, and salmon

Cereals

Look for

- Cereals that are high in fiber: whole-grain or 100% bran. Aim for products with a minimum of 3 to 4 grams of fiber per serving
- Oatmeal

Watch for

- Cereal with dried fruits and nuts, which can bump up its **PointsPlus®** value
- Added sugar and salt
- Granola, including varieties that are low in fat, which tend to have a high **PointsPlus** value

Tips

- Skip the flavored versions of oatmeal that have added sugar in the form of dried fruit. Instead, use plain oatmeal, cook it with milk, and add chopped fresh fruit such as apples or pears, blueberries, banana, etc. Your creamy oatmeal will keep you satisfied longer for a similar **PointsPlus** value
- Don't want to give up your favorite sweetened cereal with nuts? Halve your usual serving and combine it with 100% bran cereal for a lower **PointsPlus** value, more fiber, and the flavor you want

Frozen Foods

Look for

- Healthier frozen entrées, such as vegetarian burgers, entrées that feature vegetables and whole grains, and entrées without creamy sauces
- Frozen fruits and vegetables
- Low-fat or fat-free ice creams and sorbets

Watch for

- Frozen entrées high in fat, saturated fat, and sodium, such as pizza, tacos, burritos, and macaroni and cheese

Tips

- Double-bag frozen fruits and vegetables in freezer-safe bags to prolong storage and reduce freezer burn
- When comparing nutrition labels, make sure you're also looking at serving size
- Buy vegetables and fruits in loose-pack plastic bags, which make it easy to take only the amount you need

Aisle-by-Aisle Shopping Guide

Snacks

Look for

- 94% fat-free microwave or air-popped popcorn
- High-fiber whole-grain cereal bars

Watch for

- Highly processed snacks that have added sugars
- 100-calorie snacks: They may seem like a good option in terms of their **PointsPlus**® value, but they often fail to hold off hunger
- Chips and pretzels, which tend to be high in sodium and calories and low in nutrition; they won't keep you satisfied for long

Tips

- Best snacks include a combination of whole-grain carbs, protein, and some healthy fat. Try hummus with baby carrots, salsa with jicama sticks, baked corn tortillas with fat-free salsa, or a small banana or apple with a tablespoon of peanut butter
- Buy single-serving items for greater portion control. If multiple-serving-size packages are on sale, portion them out into resealable snack bags as soon as you get home

Peanut Butter, Jams, and Condiments

Look for

- Natural varieties of peanut butter
- All-fruit spreads with no added sugar, sweetened with juice
- Light or fat-free versions of mayonnaise
- Mustard

Watch for

- Added ingredients in peanut butter, such as oil, salt, and sugar
- Jams and jellies with little fruit that list sugar or high-fructose corn syrup high on the ingredients list

Tips

- Try combination mustard-and-mayonnaise spreads for more flavor and less fat than mayonnaise alone

Breads and Bakery

Look for

- 100% whole-grain products where the first ingredient listed is a whole grain, such as whole wheat or oatmeal
- Choices with 3 g fiber or more per serving
- Mini bagels made with 100% whole wheat
- Angel food cake, or reduced-fat versions of cakes
- Bread products enriched with B vitamins, iron, and folic acid

Watch for

- Large bagels made with white flour, especially those with added sugar
- Higher-fat items like muffins, croissants, doughnuts, and sweet rolls

Tips

- Stick to reduced-calorie versions of whole-grain breads for the lowest *PointsPlus*® value
- Use your weekly *PointsPlus* Allowance for the occasional doughnut or muffin treat

Baking

Look for

- Whole-wheat flour
- Flour made from grains such as corn (made from finely ground cornmeal), triticale, and oats
- Reduced-fat versions of baking mixes

Watch for

- Baking mixes with added nuts and/or extra chocolate

Tips

- When a cake calls for eggs, reduce the fat and **PointsPlus** value by substituting egg whites or egg substitute for whole eggs
- When baking brownies and cake from mixes, cut the fat in half by substituting half the called-for oil or butter with applesauce

Ethnic Foods

Look for

- Whole-grain varieties of Asian noodles, such as soba noodles made from buckwheat
- Corn and whole-wheat tortillas
- Fat-free refried beans
- Salsas without added fat
- Reduced-sodium versions of teriyaki, chili, and soy sauces

Watch for

- Microwavable prepared rice mixes, which usually have added fat and salt
- Flour tortillas, which typically have more calories and less fiber than corn tortillas
- Entrées, soups, or sauces with regular coconut milk, which is high in saturated fat
- Dried noodle soups and entrées, which are typically high in fat and sodium

Tips

- Halve the seasoning packet included in ethnic rice mixes or soups
- When mixes call for oil, use lemon juice or low-sodium vegetable or chicken broth instead

Notes

Like picking up ideas in your meetings?
Here, write down the grocery items you want to try.

_____

_____

_____

_____

_____

_____

_____

_____

_____

_____

_____

_____

_____

_____

_____

Use the foods on this list to create weight-loss-friendly Spaces in your kitchen

Pantry
List

Some of the foods listed on these pages are Weight Watchers Power Foods. Just look for the pyramid.

Pantry List

Canned Goods

▲ Beans, canned (rinse before using to lower sodium)

▲ Salmon, canned in water

▲ Tomatoes, canned, reduced-sodium, diced/plum/stewed

▲ Tuna, canned in water (light has less mercury than white or albacore)

Vegetable soups, canned, reduced-sodium

Condiments and Seasonings

Artificial sweetener

Dried herbs and spices

Ketchup

Mayonnaise, fat-free

Mustard

Vinegars, flavored

Grains and Nuts

▲ Cereals, whole grain, ready-to-eat fortified (no added sugar, dried fruits, or nuts)

Croutons

Nuts (chopped walnuts, sliced almonds, pine nuts)

▲ Oatmeal (cooked)

Tortilla chips, baked, low-fat

▲ Whole grains:
  ▲ Brown rice
  ▲ Brown rice pasta
  ▲ Bulgur
  ▲ Quinoa
  ▲ Whole-wheat pasta
  ▲ Wild rice

Tip

Weight Watchers eTools subscribers: For more ideas about shopping and planning for a well-stocked kitchen, click on the Food & Recipes tab.

Oils, Sauces, and Spreads

Barbecue sauce (reduced-sodium if available)

Oils:

    Canola

    Flaxseed

    Olive

    Safflower

    Sunflower

Pasta sauce, jarred or canned (lower sodium if available)

Peanut butter, reduced-fat

Pesto sauce, reduced-fat

Salad dressings, fat-free or light

▲ Salsa, fat-free

Soy sauce, reduced-sodium

Steak sauce (reduced-sodium if available)

Teriyaki sauce, reduced-sodium

▲ Tomato sauce, canned, reduced-sodium

Pantry List

Turn here to determine the activity *PointsPlus*® values you earn through exercise.

Activity *PointsPlus* Value Charts

You earn activity **PointsPlus** values for activity that's above your normal, everyday movements. To determine your earned activity **PointsPlus** values, you just need your current weight, the number of minutes you've exercised, and the intensity level.

Activity
PointsPlus
Value
Charts

Determining Your Intensity Level

To determine your intensity level, use your own rating
of perceived exertion (RPE):

Can you talk?	Can you sing?	Is your breathing...	Are you sweating?	Intensity level
Yes	Yes	Regular?	No	Low
Yes	No	Often and deep?	After 10 minutes	Moderate
Briefly	No	Rapid and deep?	After 3–5 minutes	High

Minutes	10			15			20		
Weight lbs	L	M	H	L	M	H	L	M	H
100	0	0	1	0	1	2	1	1	2
110	0	1	1	1	1	2	1	1	3
120	0	1	1	1	1	2	1	1	3
130	0	1	2	1	1	2	1	1	3
140	0	1	2	1	1	2	1	1	3
150	0	1	2	1	1	3	1	1	3
160	1	1	2	1	1	3	1	1	4
170	1	1	2	1	1	3	1	2	4
180	1	1	2	1	1	3	1	2	4
190	1	1	2	1	1	3	1	2	4
200	1	1	2	1	1	3	1	2	5
210	1	1	2	1	1	4	1	2	5
220	1	1	3	1	2	4	1	2	5
230	1	1	3	1	2	4	2	2	5
240	1	1	3	1	2	4	2	2	6
250	1	1	3	1	2	4	2	2	6
260	1	1	3	1	2	5	2	2	6
270	1	1	3	1	2	5	2	2	6
280	1	1	3	1	2	5	2	3	6
290	1	1	3	1	2	5	2	3	7
300	1	1	3	1	2	5	2	3	7
310	1	1	4	2	2	5	2	3	7
320	1	1	4	2	2	6	2	3	7
330	1	2	4	2	2	6	2	3	8
340	1	2	4	2	2	6	2	3	8
350	1	2	4	2	2	6	2	3	8

L Low intensity   M Moderate intensity   H High intensity

Minutes	25			30			35		
Weight lbs	L	M	H	L	M	H	L	M	H
100	1	1	3	1	1	3	1	2	4
110	1	1	3	1	2	4	1	2	4
120	1	1	3	1	2	4	1	2	5
130	1	1	4	1	2	5	2	2	5
140	1	2	4	1	2	5	2	2	6
150	1	2	4	1	2	5	2	2	6
160	1	2	5	2	2	6	2	3	6
170	1	2	5	2	2	6	2	3	7
180	1	2	5	2	2	6	2	3	7
190	2	2	5	2	3	7	2	3	8
200	2	2	6	2	3	7	2	3	8
210	2	2	6	2	3	7	2	3	8
220	2	3	6	2	3	8	3	4	9
230	2	3	7	2	3	8	3	4	9
240	2	3	7	2	3	8	3	4	10
250	2	3	7	2	3	9	3	4	10
260	2	3	8	3	4	9	3	4	11
270	2	3	8	3	4	9	3	4	11
280	2	3	8	3	4	10	3	5	11
290	2	3	8	3	4	10	3	5	12
300	2	3	9	3	4	10	3	5	12
310	3	4	9	3	4	11	4	5	13
320	3	4	9	3	4	11	4	5	13
330	3	4	10	3	5	11	4	5	13
340	3	4	10	3	5	12	4	5	14
350	3	4	10	3	5	12	4	6	14

*Instructions can be found in *Frequently Asked Questions*.

Activity *PointsPlus*® Value Charts

Minutes	40			45			50		
Weight lbs	L	M	H	L	M	H	L	M	H
100	1	2	5	1	2	5	2	2	6
110	1	2	5	2	2	6	2	3	6
120	2	2	6	2	2	6	2	3	7
130	2	2	6	2	3	7	2	3	8
140	2	3	6	2	3	7	2	3	8
150	2	3	7	2	3	8	2	3	9
160	2	3	7	2	3	8	3	4	9
170	2	3	8	3	4	9	3	4	10
180	2	3	8	3	4	9	3	4	10
190	3	4	9	3	4	10	3	4	11
200	3	4	9	3	4	10	3	5	12
210	3	4	10	3	4	11	3	5	12
220	3	4	10	3	5	11	4	5	13
230	3	4	11	3	5	12	4	5	13
240	3	4	11	4	5	12	4	6	14
250	3	5	12	4	5	13	4	6	14
260	3	5	12	4	5	14	4	6	15
270	4	5	12	4	6	14	4	6	16
280	4	5	13	4	6	15	5	6	16
290	4	5	13	4	6	15	5	7	17
300	4	6	14	4	6	16	5	7	17
310	4	6	14	5	6	16	5	7	18
320	4	6	15	5	7	17	5	7	18
330	4	6	15	5	7	17	5	8	19
340	4	6	16	5	7	18	6	8	20
350	5	6	16	5	7	18	6	8	20

L Low intensity   M Moderate intensity   H High intensity

Minutes	55			60		
Weight lbs	L	M	H	L	M	H
100	2	3	6	2	3	7
110	2	3	7	2	3	8
120	2	3	8	2	3	8
130	2	3	8	3	4	9
140	3	4	9	3	4	10
150	3	4	10	3	4	10
160	3	4	10	3	4	11
170	3	4	11	3	5	12
180	3	5	11	4	5	12
190	3	5	12	4	5	13
200	4	5	13	4	6	14
210	4	5	13	4	6	15
220	4	6	14	4	6	15
230	4	6	15	5	6	16
240	4	6	15	5	7	17
250	5	6	16	5	7	17
260	5	7	17	5	7	18
270	5	7	17	5	7	19
280	5	7	18	6	8	19
290	5	7	18	6	8	20
300	5	8	19	6	8	21
310	6	8	20	6	9	21
320	6	8	20	6	9	22
330	6	8	21	7	9	23
340	6	9	22	7	9	24
350	6	9	22	7	10	24

*Instructions can be found in *Frequently Asked Questions*.

Activity *PointsPlus* Value Charts

**Attend every week
for accountability,
support, and ideas.**

Your Meeting

As you lose weight and hit your milestones, make sure your Leader knows it. That way, he or she can be sure you're getting the right rewards and can help you celebrate—either publicly or privately, whichever you prefer.

Weigh-in Advice

We've seen members cross their fingers at the scale; take off shoes, sweaters, belts; close their eyes. Whatever works for you, works for us. The following advice, however, works for everybody.

For best results at the scale

- Weigh in at the same time each week—same day and same time of day.
- After every weigh-in, record in your Weight Record what was different that week. Did you Track? Amp up your activity routine? Eat extra Weight Watchers Power Foods?

Meeting
Rewards

Sticker Rewards

When you	You get
Lose 5 pounds	**5-Pounds Sticker** You'll get another one for each 5 pounds you lose
Report a nonscale victory, or NSV, during your meeting	**BRAVO Sticker** Your Leader will recognize and reward achievements related to the development of healthy attitudes and behaviors
Lose 5% of your starting weight	**5% Sticker**

Your Meeting

Keychain Rewards

When you	You get
Lose 10% of your starting weight	**Key Ring**
Lose 25, 50, 75, and/or 100 pounds	**Circle Charms** Put them on your key ring!
Have attended 16 paid meetings	**"Stay and Succeed," or "SAS," Charm**
Achieve your ultimate weight goal, whatever your ultimate weight goal is, whether or not it's within the Healthy Weight Ranges	**Star Charm**

Lifetime Membership

When you

Finish six weeks of maintenance as a paid, current member, weighing in at least twice during that period.
After that period, as long as you weigh in within two pounds of the ultimate goal that you agree upon with your Leader—from the Healthy Weight Ranges chart in the *Weight Record*; or as defined by your physician—that is at least five pounds less than your starting weight

You get

Key Charm and Lifetime Membership
As a Lifetime Member, you'll never pay a registration fee, and as long as you weigh in monthly within two pounds of your defined ultimate weight goal, meetings are free of charge. We'll continue to reward you—with stickers and additional charms—for continued attendance within two pounds of your weight goal.

Your Meeting

Lifetime Membership Rewards

When you	You get
Attend your first meeting of the month, weighing in within 2 pounds of your weight goal	BRAVO sticker to acknowledge your monthly attendance at goal
Have collected 10 out of 12 attendance stickers in a year	Another keychain reward for your keychain

Place your BRAVO rewards stickers here

Your Meeting

Place your BRAVO rewards stickers here

Your Meeting

Lifetime Members, place your monthly attendance stickers here

Collect 10 per year for a Keychain Reward

month _____

month _____

month _____

month _____

month _____

month _____